REFLECTIONS ON LIFE

Christopher Ejsmond

Christopher Ejsmond

All rights reserved, no part of this publication may be reproduced by any means, electronic, mechanical photocopying, documentary, film or in any other format without prior written permission of the publisher.

>
> Published by
> Chipmunkapublishing
> PO Box 6872
> Brentwood
> Essex CM13 1ZT
> United Kingdom

http://www.chipmunkapublishing.com

Copyright © Christopher Ejsmond 2008

Chipmunkapublishing gratefully acknowledges the support of Arts Council England.

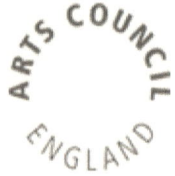

REFLECTIONS ON LIFE

A Lesson in Life

Many people will tell you that they're your friend
Till the time comes that you need them and they turn away
Do you really need them and the signals they send?
Like me, they only have two hands to lend

One day the path that you tread will crumble
And all around you will begin to fall apart
The mountain side will be steep
And time will not be on your side to keep

As the moments tick by
You'd better look out for any reason why
You should stay to receive some wisdom
And know that sometimes it's wiser to watch than to leap

Christopher Ejsmond

A walk along the tracks

As I walked along the parallel lines
In a forbidden land beyond the confines
I wanted to be there in ages past
And draw me near to the stationary mast

Human traces are left behind in strange places
Their faces no longer visible to the eye
But their thoughts and actions are still there
Trained to see in the darkness of the wild side

The tracks called me to the other side
Of the bridge
The sun did not shine on this long day
All was bathed in supernatural light

I ventured forth, my life in my hands
Amid the fury and tumultuous plans
Of the sacred railway lands
And their forgotten secrets to be told

I was the chosen one
A pioneer on a distant shore
Where no-one had ever trodden before
And no-one had dared to confront the call of the wild winds that blow down

Of human frailty I know this much
That sometimes it is better to ponder than to touch
And that when others turn their backs
You will find me walking along the railway tracks

REFLECTIONS ON LIFE

Angels

I sat in the dried up river bed
Alive for now but almost dead
Broken bottles strewn all around
And empty cans of lager on the ground
Broken trees and sloping concrete sides
A hot summer's day was the measure of time

What was I doing there, in that desperate land?
Connecting to everything through the sublime hand
The light was fantastic
Visionary mind which faltered and took action drastic
The air was still and there was no sound
Then came the angels just before I drowned

They offered me protection
From my own psychic affliction
Connected they were by a silver thread
Wings they had and in harmony they said
That I would be safe in their hands
As they delivered me from these strange lands

Before my very eyes, I knew that they did exist
How futile it was their message of hope to resist
Since then I have been watching for their return every day
Hoping that they're coming back – I'll send them not away
I'm seeing all the signs and learning how to bring them back

Christopher Ejsmond

Forever waiting for the angels to return and set me on their track

And deliver once more that glimpse of the other world
Before I die of fright and somewhere else I turn
What will I know in that moment of ecstasy?
One day they will come back and deliver their promise to me
O spectacle of light, vision extraordinaire
Spare me not forever your divine presence, I know not how, I know not where

REFLECTIONS ON LIFE

Birdsong in spring

The trap is set
These words I pen lest I forget
The mind is weak
What is it that I seek?

The sound of the bird in innocent flight
The clamour of song with enlightened sight
The churlish menace from without
Engulfs all my senses and churns me out

The light in spring is a wonderful thing
The blackbird sings as it flaps its wings
Yet I die amid the turmoil of life
To be reborn – a new man, a new face
And in another place

Christopher Ejsmond

Breaking the Rules

I have lived my life in the shadows of the rule makers
But now I have joined the ranks of the rule breakers
Together we challenge the social conspiracy
For we are the mutilated ones left adrift by society

We stand apart from the rest of you
It's no one's fault that you know not what to do
Or how to react when things go wrong
Escape, if you can, from the motley throng

Flock not to the shadowy depths
For there is nothing there for you but the sorrows of those who have wept
And flooded the land with their silver tears
As others stand idly by and raise their cheers

Your rules are meant to be broken
The secret code which worked so well is now but an empty token
Of one of life's greatest mysteries
Which to this day locks us away in our miseries

This life is still worth living
Even if the deceitful rules seem unforgiving
For who in this world has stopped to ask us
Or shown mercy for our freedoms which you seek to truss

How much longer must we suffer this indignity?

REFLECTIONS ON LIFE

And when will the final healing restore us from your ignominy?
If we are ever to fully lead our lives freely
Then we must all learn to break these social rules unreservedly

Christopher Ejsmond

Complications

You shine a light into the dark corners of my mind
What is it that you want to know?
You never let go, even when I sleep
And you search for the answer to a question unasked
Why do you seek to complicate life?
And how will you know when the task is done?

I am as transparent as the air you breathe
Weak and weary of your torments
Yet I persist in the tiring onslaught
Of your unforgiving taunts
And detrimental complications
Which turn me inside out

Mine is the other life which you seek to undo
And set free the spirits of the afterlife
Yours is the unhappy invective tirade
A critical glance in my direction
Which watches me gleefully as I tire
Amid your complicated and self satisfied gestures

I know that one day I will vanquish these unwanted emotions
And live a life full of sweetness
Without your confused complications
And go forth with joy in my heart
Where the grass is greener and the sun does shine
Upon that which is rightly and truly mine

REFLECTIONS ON LIFE

Crossing The Threshold

Once I told a lie to get by
And found that all was not as it seemed
Then the dawn broke
And called across to me
It all happened in a flash of inspiration
When the lights were turned off and you sought my attention

Spurious prejudicial factors
Engage weak minds
And take them by both hands
To where people from the Steppe cross the river
They seek others to charge with conceit
And purvey the horizon of deceit

When I cross over to the other side
I want to learn from the pressure pushing down on me
And take me to a place far away from here
Where the morning air is clean
And where others serve in the shadows of the occultation
Of the starry messenger's celestial mediation

I'd like to know
Just how strong you really are
So that I may jest about the barbaric side
Resistance is futile
And soon I will emerge cleansed by the torture
Of the chamber where dwells the evil creature

When I cross the threshold of despair

Christopher Ejsmond

I am taken to the place of the armed warriors
And take my place among the legions
Whereby all is transposed by eternal correlation
And the magical place sings on in my heart
That one day I may at last my life to start

REFLECTIONS ON LIFE

Don't Look Now

In a place far away there is a cavern
Where the night brings new life to fathom
A door shuts and another one opens
On the inner world of dreams and self abandon

This is a place where past meets present
And things dark seem at once so pleasant
Unless they bear a sinister tone
Of angels which have long since flown

It's happened before and it will happen again
I've followed the path through shrewd acumen
To ask, perhaps, whether we are mad when we dream
Or just as sane as the rest, so it would seem

Don't look now for you will not like what you see
Only I can appreciate this molecular level of reality
And only I can tell you where I end and the world begins
For it is my life you will see amid the monumental ruins

Christopher Ejsmond

Echoland

. . . standing alone, frozen and motionless
Listening to the birds sing in the trees
And piecing together the decree of my own naivety
Of the things I do hear all around
I walk on and I am transmuted
By the echoes of the borderland

Travelling on buses in the dusk
Through dusty lands and islands of traffic
I see through the wastelands where the vagrant abides
On this forgotten side of life
Amid the detritus of the rotting souls on the forgotten side
And the echoes of the nether land

A door slams in the distance
A child cries out for its mother
The lamenting metallic drone of the aeroplane overhead
And the shriek of the siren
All is sound now and wasted not
In the echoes of the hinterland

The menace of repeated sound cascades down
And turns me inside out
Delivering me to the other side again
Waiting for my return
To successive recurrence
With the echoes of the echoland . . .

REFLECTIONS ON LIFE

Edge of Madness

I was standing on the brow of a hill
Looking down on the benign rows of dwellings
The air was cold and damp
The sun did not shine; it just lingered on in the sky

Then I turned to you and asked you why
When the light begins to fade, there is stillness in the air
And the birds sing no more but seek their nests
As we walked on, the shadows danced and embraced the night

I was in distress; it didn't matter on the company
The winter light faded fast and my heart beated loudly
I was on the edge of another place and time
And playing the waiting game

Waiting for the men in white coats to appear
And take me far away from here
Where the sun never shines
And nature's old felicities to meet

Moved by the unconquerable mind
I plunged ever deeper into that despair
From which there is no return
Intoxicated by the very same air that you breathe

The sun had long ago descended in the west
And the evening star did indeed shine
On me, standing here at the edge of madness

Christopher Ejsmond

Where no-one dares to go but I, enthused by its tenderness

REFLECTIONS ON LIFE

Father, dear father

You never had time for me
You drank away my happiest years
You never listened to a word I said
What you wanted was never made clear
Behind the façade was ignorance and fear

You walked behind in the shadows of the great ones
And still followed the same old path of self-destruction
I'm not sure when began your infidelity
I won't be treated as your property

You never stayed at home too long
Not once did you ask me what was wrong
I don't think you ever really cared
With glib and deceitful delight you hung on to the opinions of others who were stronger
But now I know that there are two sides to every story
And surely, somebody had to help me

I still see it in your eyes
Wasn't it a tragedy?
The silence in your eyes
Betrayed the storms beneath the oceanic currents

In the name of the father, I will not give in
You will find me all alone now
I'm only sorry that I stayed too long
I never realised that at one time it was you that did
I idolize

Christopher Ejsmond

Whatever I intended, you thwarted and undid
Made me weak and wish that I could start all over again

Your punitive hands were strong in those days
But you're a stranger to me now
You tried to teach me things I didn't need to know
But life is too short to be afraid
It should be clear by now that my entrance into this world was of my own creation
And that now I should take the praise, while you suffer in your frustration

I still blame you for the way things turned out to be
For running round in circles and plunged into this life of dismal solitude
You fell from grace long ago and now I depend on so-called friends
It's a pity that in those days you needed to hide in your defence

Some of your ways you just couldn't mend
For I remember them all, those fragile days!
Strange little man! It didn't take long for me to find out that I had enough

Today you will find me controlled in the body and controlled in the mind
Too busy fighting the slavish mindset which you helped in me to bind
My life belongs to me now, even though you made me feel ashamed of you

REFLECTIONS ON LIFE

For I've got the stars on my side, while you sit and suffer for your lies and for what you failed to do
What can you expect to be said in confidence?
It was someone who used you so well that had the last laugh

Christopher Ejsmond

Flashback

I saw you standing there
On the subterranean pathway
A place so dark and yet so full of light
To show the way to the other world

I know what this life does mean to me
From the depths of despair have I cried
The gathering harvest is now upon us
And the remnants of summer fade away

I remember those days well
When the revelation of all our yesterdays came
And delivered the promise of hope
Upon life's journey to I know not where

Bright colours and newly born light
Amid strange sounds of the birds in full song

Those were truly the acid days
And my soul was nourished from within
If all else is left in doubt
Then I am the last man standing
On life's great roundabout of sorrow and forgiveness

REFLECTIONS ON LIFE

Friendship

All that I am
All that I ever was
Is here in your perfect eyes
They're all I can see

A love broken in two
Like it never was
Alone now in a desolate world
Only memories to nurse my wounds

Before I can smile and laugh again
I know I need to see your perfect eyes
If ever I am to recover that which I once was
Together once more we must be
Together once more we must be

Christopher Ejsmond

Golden age

Before I became who I am today
In a time so distant, so long ago
Before the days turned into the longest of dark nights
I came into this world one golden autumn's day

Golden years they surely were
But they went quickly by
Pure and immortal then I was
The heavens moved around me in perpetual dance

All was harmony and peace within
This inceptual phase did wax and wane
The paradigm was never lost
And the sweetness of time bore fruit

I lived like a god without sorrow of heart
Blessed by the abundance of peace and light
In the beginning was this ideal state
Which did end with my falling asleep

When it ceased to be I was thrust into the all-consuming fires of madness
Prometheus was now truly unbound
And Pandora opened her treasure chest to all around
But now a new age of legends beckons

REFLECTIONS ON LIFE

Grief Reaction

The big question is hard to handle
But when you left it was a greater scandal
In the church of the Holy Family your body did lay
Serene and surreal, for someone who could not pray

Life left your body and your soul departed
The women wept and were left broken hearted
Hoping for a revelation
But instead there was consternation

Your refusal to attend the sacraments and Christian duties
They understood not why you so valued your own liberties
And what promise of eternal life
Could bear down on you in the afterlife?

After you went, I found God again
And learned how to trust in the final amen
I joined the reverential ones
And the life of the spirit had truly begun

I became a catalyst in your last requiem
Of binding words and solemn deeds I did not condemn
A Son of God, a priest to be, at last, safe from sin
Dignity in loss which I could win

Forgiving to the last
And surrendered to Papal infallibility I was cast

Christopher Ejsmond

There was no Extreme Unction; it was not your request
Against rite and ritual you continued to protest

REFLECTIONS ON LIFE

Heroes

The sun vanishes from the sky
And touches their golden skin
The rivers freeze over
And the wind does blow down again
On unsung heroes in the field of the giants
Where they stand and receive new life
From the electric dance of the atom
Never at rest, its depths to fathom

Where will it end, this magnetic chorus
Of angels and demons
Of dwarves and giants?
And how will they call you if they know not your name
From among the masses whence you came?

The sun revolves around you
And the bond of innocence is broken
Sweet melodies ring forth to embrace the day
While the same sad song does play
You are never truly alone now
Your fame speaks to the nations
About your ecstatic lamentations
And heroic expectations

Christopher Ejsmond

He's Been Away

Get back to your ward behind the palatial façade
And run back to your closed world
Forgive those who would harm your mind
And poison your body with medication
For you have known true sorrow
Alone you have stood up to the world when all around were in darkness

The social landscape of the asylum is where you have been until now
Too afraid to go out of the door, you cower and bend your head in shame
You've been away, locked in a padded cell
Exorcised by doctors who knew best at the time
Optimistic that one day you would recover your sanity
And stand at the margins of care in the community

You are one of the long stay patients
Resettled for now until another crisis descends upon you
The prospects don't look good
And your fortunes have run out of time
You sit there motionless watching television
That's worse for your health than hospital admission

Rejected by society, you struggle to survive
And face the crowds of the new pessimism
It's not your fault that you have chosen loneliness
Experience has shown that there are no true friends out there

REFLECTIONS ON LIFE

The stigma is real and a painful cut
Into the wounded flesh that no longer heals

You are now part of the new debate
Partners in healthcare and now you have a voice of your own
Although you have set foot on new horizons as a 'user'
You find yourself back at the bottom of the pile
Not a full member of your community
But a nameless statistic whereby others react to your illness

The services are limited and your 'involvement' sparse
Yet you have grown in strength even though you have been forgotten
By unethical considerations
And foreboding mental health proclamations
One day, perhaps, you will surely find
That broken though you are, you are still a person with a name

Christopher Ejsmond

Hospital

Places of sickness nurse me cold
As the stale air does gently unfold
Tying me to the dreary routines of this altered life
Medicated, sedated I lie there
Waiting to be told that it's alright
Now to go home
And behold
The splendours of the outside world

REFLECTIONS ON LIFE

I can see for miles

I can see for miles and miles
Beyond the horizon, where sky meets sea
I can fly for hours and hours
Beneath the celestial key

Which open the doors of paradise
To welcome the weary stranger
And beckons him to enjoin
And turn his back on danger

As the light fades and the birds seek their final place of rest
I stretch out my hand and touch the sky
Where sky meets sea, I endeavour to be
At rest at last with the angels on high

Christopher Ejsmond

I wish I could fly

I wish I could fly
And soar high into the velvet sky
Like a seagull or an eagle
I would descend from a steeple

If only I could fly
As I do in dreams
High above the fields of corn
And higher than the Matterhorn

I wish I could fly
But instead surrender to a sigh
Abide by me, oh heavens above
And deliver my soul to the spiritual dove

REFLECTIONS ON LIFE

If you fear you're losing me

If you fear you're losing me
Remember I've returned to the sanctuary
Where I'll give them my finest hour
And return to you with super human power

I hear you spend the night time crying
While others around you are deceitfully lying
Waiting for the time when you're too weak
To call for help and remedy seek

It's all a mystery
Part of my destiny
Hidden voices mock my words
And electric faces seem to merge

Dreams become reality
And no-one knows my hidden frailty
They simply look away
And find solace in another day

The very young need the sun
To bring peace of mind when all else is said and done
And now, my friend, I must return to the world of my dreams
For that is all there is, or so it seems

In between the adorable delusion
Lies the hidden and incurable confusion
It seemed like the real thing
The promise of the other world I thought it would bring

Christopher Ejsmond

Then I realised that no-one was listening
Yet your eyes told me that I was hastening
And when all the lights went finally out
I plunged ever deeper into that misery and doubt

Then the day came when it fell from me like an avalanche
And I found myself embraced in that familiar magical dance
Was this madness divine or merely sublimely unfurled?
And will it come to pass again in another world?

REFLECTIONS ON LIFE

In dreams

Many of my dreams are about the past
Sometimes they call my name
Others run by or speed up too fast
Blasting me apart, never to remain the same

Some of my dreams are about what is to pass
A running commentary from inside
Bringing forth the promise of secret knowledge
And leaving nowhere for me to hide

Christopher Ejsmond

In God did I trust

When I found you, o my God
It was like a bolt out of the blue
For I knew in that moment what it was I had to do
The world of symbols came to life once more
And no longer was I a mere pebble on a deserted shore

In the moment of that revelation
My mind was freed at last from its languishing perturbation
I saw you for who you truly are
Blessed by your promise that you were never very far

I bore my cross with utmost dignity
Surrendered my soul to the Blessed Trinity
The secret knowledge was a special thing
I truly believed in you, that you were my king

I fell to my knees in that hour of need
Enraptured by your recognition, I followed your creed
I saw the gates of paradise open before me
I gave in to your total supremacy

I moved with you as a child seeking parental affection
A tender perfection which took me in a new direction
The angels were truly on my side
I was a soldier of Christ; no longer did I need to hide

REFLECTIONS ON LIFE

I learnt to forgive and to restore my faith
You made me feel that life was worth living again
and that the journey would be safe
The Promised Land was here indeed
I praised you o Lord for planting this seed

You were my spiritual nemesis
But you were also my undoing
For just as I had found you in my desolation
So I learnt to despise you, o great destroyer of civilizations

In YOUR name did they not level the great cities of the Incas?
And did they not also destroy the sacred Baltic oaks?
Did not the blood of nations run through their fingers?
Perfidious tyrants for whom frail humanity was but a bad joke

I tire of you, o Popes and Potentates
The layers of your bloody history suffocate the unborn
And subject the innocents to the stain of original sin
While damning the reputations of those long since gone

You would have us all as your obedient slaves
Perverted Christianity, you call all those 'others' infidels

Christopher Ejsmond

Blinded by your own vanity, you crown your princes
A crime against humanity, which no longer convinces

Come down from your heights o men of God
Come out of your churches and smell the blood of your wrath
The detritus of your martyrdom decays among the unholy ones
Your churlish sacraments sit uncomfortably among the suffering children who play in the sun

Imported lies and virginal frustrations
Follow the hypocrisy and the path of destiny
Your soldiers and warriors who went before your dignitaries
Paid the highest price of all, higher than your devoted signatories

Today, we all pay for the bribery
We are all the slaves of our own history
The long pilgrimage is over
And the enigmatic lies at last uncovered

How do you set the limits on your liability?
Resurrection? There is none. Only the certainty of your own accountability
The mockery of insincere complications
Is the vacillation of falsification

Life after death? There is none.
The nails used to bind you to the cross have won

REFLECTIONS ON LIFE

Crowned and crucified, you still look down on us in contempt and sorrow
And repose in the electric untouchable glow of your incarnate furrows

I am not, nor ever could be part of your body
I don't need you any more, o vanquished visionary
Stand no longer in my way – release the battered children from their purgatory
For I have no faith in you and have rendered apart the binding chains of my self-declared blasphemy

Christopher Ejsmond

July 1972

You did what you did when you wanted to
Because you knew you could
You exposed me to your world of want and need
You were old
I was only a child barely out of my mother's tender embrace
You didn't care how got what you wanted from me
You don't even remember my face

I cried out for mercy
But instead you inflicted the pain I still remember today
You've taken everything away
You made me the way I am today
Forever lost to your vile design
Forever the handmaiden of secrecy and deception
I grew up before my time

You had this idea from the confusion of your soul
You still took when you knew I had given it all
You hung on to me
For you held the key
And the final decision wasn't up to me
Tell me that I'm dreaming for I want to live
And I'll tell you that you're the seedy one who I can't forgive

Tell me why I'm being sucked dry
I don't need this display of affection
And I certainly don't appreciate your type of protection
Am I just another piece of paper in your file?

REFLECTIONS ON LIFE

How could I trust you, wretched paedophile?

Strip me bare
Colour me in
Rub me out
I promise not to shout
Rip my body to shreds
Re-arrange my mind!
Show me desire – but one that's not mine

Your generous genitals – tangential sex
Totally unethical and fruitless waste
You seek to destroy that which is innocent
And you have no regrets
You remain in the clear – a pillar of respect!

Extinguish any trace of humanity
As you fondle me divergently
Your lust and greed I do not need
Contamination through masturbation!
You tasted me then you wasted me

More than I want to, more than I can
I had no-one to turn to then when I needed to cry
You had no shame
When you played that filthy game
And now?
Gone are those days and gone is the time you took away from me

You had me where you wanted me
You rode over me
And you sucked my energy

Christopher Ejsmond

You took me in your wretched arms when I was still a child
You taught me to lie and not to confide
By showing me that this is yours and that is mine

You've got your own history and time to back up YOUR claims
You inflicted pain on my tortured body and tormented my mind
Not to mention all my loss – I had from YOU no gains, but chains
You sought to protect your own future happiness and security
Amid my inner turmoil what happiness could that child find?

I was a victim of your sordid oppression
And now I wake to that dull and grey depression
Alone I sleep in fear and with emotions frayed
I was weaker once but now I'm stronger and better than you could ever be

You used me as a tool
Treated me like a fool
Fucked me up
Mucked me up
Treated me like a toy
Something to destroy

Fucked up – totally
Mucked up – permanently
Totally abused
Utterly bemused
Pulled about

REFLECTIONS ON LIFE

Fooled about
You're the one to blame
But I don't need your games

Christopher Ejsmond

Life after sunset

The sun sets on the longest day
When all the world's sorrows have passed away
Together now we stand before the night
To witness an angel in perfect flight

My heart pounds, my head spins
My mind is full of the darkest of things
Yet your presence lifts my soul to eternal joy
As I lay down before you, exhausted by toil

REFLECTIONS ON LIFE

Life Cycles

Organized complexity resides in all systems
Where human beings are involved
Groups of objects work in concert to produce a given result
And the cycle of life marches onwards

Cognitive deficits are ontological aberrations
Which are modified by behavioural traits
And emotional susceptibility
However, the whole is more than the sum of its parts

Emergent properties offer analogues for living systems
And attribute nomenclatural reference points
To paradigms lost to the human life cycle
Interdependent in the extreme analysis

And so the key to life's mysteries is found
Elements in isolation we are not
But depend on one another
Connected by a mysterious web of constituent relationships

Christopher Ejsmond

London Bridge station (Journey to Bethlem)

Leaving for Bethlem was the hardest thing of all
I journeyed there high above the ground on great arches and brick walls
From London Bridge station
To this place of the incurables, my final destination

The faded grandeur of the terminus drew far behind into the distance
Its mysterious underground caverns held on with benign persistence
From the blind corners of the secret cathedral with lotus leaf capital
To the strange land behind a wall in setting pastoral

As I entered the orchard of the Monks
Iron grating and bars I witnessed not amid the detritus and junk
Instead, the warm red brick of this ancient villa did I see
And the décor of the third decade did speak to me

Raving and Melancholy Madness stood to one side
And the men and women whose minds had been seized did hide
Their human stories, one by one, they proclaimed
And the instruments of restraint did they blame

The iron manacle rules here no more
And the strait waistcoat is discarded and no longer in store

REFLECTIONS ON LIFE

Polite society no longer makes sport and diversion
Of the inhabitants in their state of pathological conversion

This birdcage of care and control
Has witnessed how the thousands who did once enrol
Their chains of descent to diagnostic label
Distress and recovery do now engage in this Tower of Babel

Today, they study not the physiognomy of insanity
But prefer to image the brain for greater clarity
The Basketmen have at last found their voice
And, enlightened, promote freedom of choice

Christopher Ejsmond

Loneliness

Alone at last with head held high
A solitary figure with nowhere to run
With no-one to love and nothing to hide
Alone in the world when all is done
When all is done, all is done

REFLECTIONS ON LIFE

Lost At Sea

The tide was high and the sky was blood red
I had lost my way and was feared for dead
On that long day before I wept
And called out to you as you slept

All was forgiven, the slights and insults
For I had known you in better times before the hunt
Of the wild horses tamed on the golden plain
Where earth meets sea in the loss of pain

Where are you now?
I do not know how
You moved beyond the silver surf
Gracefully mourning my return

Christopher Ejsmond

Man on a white horse

I saw you ride out one day from the east
And travel on horseback to the opium den
Through the ages, you're heading west
Where an angel stands in the sun
You were never at rest
And put to the test before he who is faithful and true
And did the heavens not open
And lightning in three places strike?

You married the woman on a scarlet beast
And wept as you watched your children suffer her torments
Her demonic powers have turned your life to blight
But rest assured that her time will have its end
The wild horses you could not tame
And the ancestral voices I also do hear
As they rescue me from my sorrows
And after the tribulation of those days, the sun will fall from the sky

For a thousand years will dwell the righteous
For your angel with key and chain has slain the Beast
And the Tsars over you yield their power no more
That you may once more rebuild the Messiah of the Slavonic Nations
Satan is truly bound that he may deceive the nations no more
The dead utter their words to me, as they did to you before

REFLECTIONS ON LIFE

Renewed and redeemed I stand before the new creation
And in the distance I heard you proclaim your creed

Let final battle now commence
And let the fires of destruction cleanse away the vestiges of the unjust
Before those in whom you trust
Come to life again and witness the feast
Of the brave and faithful ones
Of the flag-bearers and the cavalry
And of the great ones who sit on the heavenly thrones
And do justice and mercy impart

Now that earth and sky fall asunder
And the Great White Throne does thunder
In knowledge go forth that the eyes like flames of fire
Penetrate the last secrets of the human heart
And that the scarlet beast rules no more
The winepress of the wrath of God is trodden
And your comprehending mind he alone knows
Go and seek Truth in the wisdom of age

In that final judgment day
Rest assured that your name will be found in the Book of Life
Walk up and your God you will see
Father of fathers, what will he say to you?
And how will he judge you
In that longest of days?
The secrets of your mind and soul he will know

Christopher Ejsmond

And deliver you up to the just cause

The storm of judgment is at last over
And thunder before you silenced
A new order is realised and all things he makes new
Disorder banished and now the New Jerusalem stands
On the ruins of many Babylons
Their former glory now an empty desolation
Their triumphs no more, amid the abandoned remains
You sing with the angels in glory and praise his name

REFLECTIONS ON LIFE

March of the 'Y' men

Under the stairs I sat in total darkness
Pilot of the great craft set in motion by electrical messages
Then I turned and witnessed a parade
Of brightly coloured figures – of Y's, and X's and hybrids, they stayed

Male and female they were
Gammatron emission and strange ratios
They leapt at me in their perpetual dance
Displaying infinite sequences and parental pairings

I could not break the magical code
This game was impossible to lose
Genetic segregation at this subtle level of reality
Nanotype regulation leading to ultimate schizotypy

Christopher Ejsmond

Maverick

Your cover is blown
And the rats have abandoned their lair
Others lie in wait
For me to ensnare
YOU wasted my life
And ended MY youth
While waiting there
For me, no doubt

Yours were the unusual gestures
Of greed and selfish delight
And yours were the wandering hands
Which in me did breed fright
And when all was said and done
I was left to pick up the pieces
Of a life wasted and undone
Too afraid to move on and live

You drank yourself into an early grave
Not too soon, be sure, for you had nothing for me to give
Life's simple beat kept pulsing on
And the life I led was not my own
For you this day do I bring
Not joy but an empty thing
To place on the shelf above the mantelpiece
And take comfort in the strong and fierce

REFLECTIONS ON LIFE

Mothers and sons

Mother dearest, you went too far
Mother, is that really you?
Thank you for being there for me
Your faltering ways I do not see
For you are indeed a friend to me

You gave me the gift of life
You comforted me in the dark of night
Who can explain this strongest of bonds?
Patient, forgiving, healing – you believe in me as I trust in you
You alone took away the tears I shed when you saw me you suffer, as you have done

You are the walking miracle
You give me a place of safety and you inhabit the highest pinnacle
Yours is the true and selfless devotion
The sacrifice and pain you have suffered for others' weaknesses
I will always remember and be there for you in your endurance

Creation has never witnessed such an incarnation
A mystery to behold, forever believing and beyond definition
The bond is without beginning or end
It grows each day; you will forever remain my friend

Christopher Ejsmond

Obelisk

Blank faces stare into space
And the noise of the traffic hums closely by
When I close my eyes, I see a white sheet
Waiting to be inscribed with words of stone

There are no words today
For they have all fled from my mind
Instead there is a sad emptiness
Of foreboding gloom and apprehension

When I close my eyes, I see a red sunrise
And know that new life is upon me
Where death had once dared to stalk
Breaking the fragile bonds of trust

Depressed by insight into my own plight
I denounced the deleterious world around
And forged a new friendship with inanimate things
That may bring a strange stability to the mind

The mute stones speak in verse
And show forth their majestic variability
While I compose one last valediction
To profess my existence and my affliction

REFLECTIONS ON LIFE

Object number one

Abandoned cranes stand rusting in the shipyard
As the song of the swallows pierces the still air
And the long winter evening draws in
To gather the workers on their homeward retreat
Where they will eat with their families
And bring new life to those abandoned by day

In God do they trust
And young they are in heart
To them belongs the future
Of metal fashioned into men
And their dreams live on
To deliver the promise of true happiness

This river of rust is all I see
As it meanders through adversity
And toils on the sleeping brain
Amid the background noise
Where I heard it on the radio
Of things which spin incandescent webs of deceit and lies

I sit alone and watch the day go by
Memories inside my head hold open the door
To the local colours of the rustic folk
Who live on the edge of town
And come together in a safe place
From time to time, in hiding from the human race

Christopher Ejsmond

On the choices I have made in life

I have taken many a turn
In life and in dreams, always seeking to return
To the place where I started from
And shelter seek from the strong

If I follow the path which leads
To where I truly wish to be
Will I stop and turn back
To the beginning of this beaten track?

Or will I follow and to fate abandon
All my wishes for the future state?
How will it end?
In a moment of glory?
And for just how long must I wait?

Undone by time and the threads of life
I walk along blindly
Waiting for the earth to open up
And consume the raging currents of my mind

REFLECTIONS ON LIFE

On the significance of quantum theory for schizophrenia

Larger objects such as the brain
Are the consequences of quantum behaviour
My existence is probable
And my condition shrouded in a cloud of uncertainty
Brain waves leap through the air
Watch out as they entwine and pair

The dance of the atoms is all there is
Set in motion and forever colliding
The laws of physics deteriorate on small scales
And the paradox of things seen and unseen pales
Waves which behave like particles
Describing the complex web of organised chaos

A schizophrenic brain exhibits wave-particle duality
Systems of interacting objects
Which affect each other reciprocally
Are the measure of reality
Neither from itself nor from another, nor from both,
Nor without a cause does anything whatever anywhere arise

Electrons form blurred clouds of probabilities around the nucleus
They surround the nucleus and other subatomic actions
And are located somewhere in space, their exact positions remaining unknown

Christopher Ejsmond

How is all this possible and how do we fathom the depths
of quantum indeterminacy?
Which makes possible the transmutation of lead into gold

The psychotic state lies in that region where brain and mind interact
And raises doubt over the question of agent responsibility
Brain chemicals and the scattering process locked in a dance of potentiality
Reveal all to the subtle mind attuned to receive wisdom
In this lies the contradiction of the very large and the very small
As we grow in wisdom as do the particles themselves

REFLECTIONS ON LIFE

Once I had a friend

It seemed like paradise
As I sat by and watched the river flow
Never-ending and winding
A silver picture that moved so slow

I'm holding on to a broken dream
Take me far away from here
Was it fate or was it destiny?
I don't know yet!
Or was it by pure chance?

Don't abandon me to YOUR pleasure
But sit by me and provide a measure
Of sanity

When I saw you in the distance
It was like seeing a portrait - a perfect vision of you
It was better than that empty room with no view

Dusty window-frames still arise
And musty odours to the memory bring a promise
It was another life then
And you made a man out of me
Now it's my turn to take you and show you the rules of MY life

I know who they are
And they know who I am
My life is an open book
I don't give up just like that

Christopher Ejsmond

You were my anchor, my hope, my salvation
Sparing me from desperate measures and self-mutilation
Now you can see just who is in this situation
And rise above in triumphant jubilation

REFLECTIONS ON LIFE

Overdose Melody

When I fell in love with you
I didn't want to hurt you with my lack of sympathy
For your own problems
Which were evident from the first day we met

I admired your words of gold
And your rich caress in your glorious arms
Together we were for a few stolen moments of bliss
Brought together by fate one night in April

Our love was strong
And it lasted long
There was some pain at first
But that did not last

I looked for sympathy but you didn't yet know
That I was unwell, even when in love
You took me by the hand and opened up a world
So sweet and charmed

Then one day I took those bitter pills
To nurse away all of my ills
For I wasn't very strong
And my nerves were frayed

I did it once before
When the tide of love glowed in my heart
And set aside my resolve
To assume a harmonious blend

The melody of self hate rang out in my heart

Christopher Ejsmond

While you were left standing alone
Entropic, hypnotic, and in a trance
My thoughts you read aloud and cried

In the belly of the beast I took solace
And accumulated a wealth of experience
I evaluated my condition
And what I saw within I hated

REFLECTIONS ON LIFE

People I know

People I know pass me by in the street
Without even saying hello
They're on a mission to impress
The neighbours

They go out of their way
To make my life a misery
By pretending that they do not know
The family

In living memory I have travelled
The road to perdition
Amid the remains of the day, I see before me
The general population

Walk boldly on with faith of heart
Stress proliferates and I do remedy seek
From those few kind souls of
The sociological imagination

Christopher Ejsmond

Poem of Remembrance

I remember a time when I was young

Thrown into the world
Amid colour and light
When all was still bright

Then the clouds came
And turned my mind
From peace and quiet
Into a tumultuous riot

No more could I stand the pain
No more could I see those lights
But instead I heard the voices in my head
Which screamed at me and wished me dead

Today I scream no more
For now I've learnt to open the door
To truth and happiness
And others have learnt how to heal
The wounds and sorrows of the past

REFLECTIONS ON LIFE

Raw

There are gaps in my life
And processes at work which I do not fully understand
But I know there to be more universal truth in single a grain of sand

I am like an empty vessel which shatters in the wind
Limited in expression and poor of speech
I stand here like the noble savage whom you beseech

My mind is a speculum, a mirror of the universe
A microcosm, a part of the greater whole
And dereliction it renders in my soul

As I walk on, an emptiness I feel inside
And the world around me is red and raw
Its melancholy quality I do endure

Christopher Ejsmond

Reflections on life

Life is a broken-winged bird that cannot fly
Battered by storms and brought down from on high
Life is a barren land of emotion
Of poisonous air and the witch's potion

Where do we turn to in our moment of grief?
And how do we seek moments of relief
From the turmoil of life and the tears of redemption
Seeing through life's sweet temptations

REFLECTIONS ON LIFE

Rooted

I am like a tree rooted in the earth
I come from far away
And stay for a day

My roots are deep
And my soul is perched high
Above the precipice

Flying high above the ground
I am in another place
And the rose blooms to adore me

I see the figure of a man in the tree
Which is caressed by the wind in the distance
And at last finds itself at rest

I am in a different level of reality
To that of the every day
With the voice of God by my side

There is sweet harmony in the land
But my mind is overloaded by useless information
I have just this moment sprung into existence

If I remain still for a while
And switch off from the flood of thoughts
I do hear the disembodied clamour of the
shattering voices

From one side, from on high
From another time and place

Christopher Ejsmond

From someone dead or alive come the secret messages

Another now is calling me
Before the emptiness abides in me
And delivers me to a place where I should not be

This tree is rooted in the soil that nourishes
And brings forth a new promise
Of words that paint a thousand pictures

It stands alone
Mighty and dejected
Just as I am in the midst of the turmoil around me

The continuum is a rare and precious gift
Which haunts the mind and makes no assumptions
About the way things must be

Suspended in mid air
The figure in the tree calls out to me
As the sun shines brightly

Layer upon layer of historical conditions
Have shaped me into the form of a tree
With my incredible shrinking brain

And now that the sun has shed its light
I bid the world goodnight
And return with joy to fight the good fight

REFLECTIONS ON LIFE

Something is calling me

Today I walk in the wilderness
Along the empty, foreboding streets
All I see is the old man standing alone in the corner
Time is running out for him, as it is for me
Nothing lasts for ever
All is overshadowed by eternal frequency

Where am I going? I do not know
How did I get there? I know not how
How many times have I been told and warned
About the melancholy dreamer who long before me once mourned?
And now I want to be there in the midst of it all

Welcome to this strange world
Where dreams come true and boundaries merge into what is left untold
Join me on this magical quest for truth and subtlety
But promise that you will not abandon me

The call of the other side is stronger than anything I have ever known
It embraces time and space and all therein sown
I seek not to apportion any blame
For I know not who is truly mad and who is sane
Surely we should all get the same chance to witness this
And burst forth with new life out of our chrysalis

Seek not to contradict this mysterious edict

Christopher Ejsmond

The message carried by the cold wind which
blows in from the east doesn't make a sound
Instead it wraps itself around
And is yours to be found

Let the calling stay with you a day, a month, a
year, a lifetime
Let the yearning pass and learn to embrace it as a
good sign
I have my eyes firmly on the ground
And as I walk on by I make no sound

Wait for the dust to blow and the rains to come
down
Wait for the lonely magnetic voices to draw you in
and turn your mind around
There have been too many tears shed in this one
life
I'm tired now; I've lost control and alas return once
more to bitter strife

But before I return to the darkness, let me take
you once more there
For in me the call lasts forever and makes
manifest I know not where
You're out of time now but I linger on
With the call of the wild ones, where I must stand
alone

REFLECTIONS ON LIFE

Standing out in the crowd

It was easy in those days
It was also quite legal
To be a drunk
For my mind was quite feeble

Every day, it seems
I went out for more
Cider, wine and spirits
Did I particularly adore

What mattered to me most
Did not arrive in the post
But was found in a bottle
As I watched the world go quietly by, I accelerated the throttle

Whenever I decided to go on a bender
It was always me who was the biggest spender
I lost sight of everything
For the few brief moments of happiness the alcohol would bring

Would I end up like the drunk sitting on the park bench
Or stand out in the crowd as I ignominiously wrench?
Raise your glasses, why don't you?
One more for the road?
And remember – Guinness is good for you!

I heard many times that it was a 'social' problem
And that no matter who, no matter when

Christopher Ejsmond

Could become another faceless statistic
In this embarrassing public health heuristic

Let us raise a toast to the spring
And to all the glory that it will bring
The innocent lunchtime drink at work
Is all that I needed to keep me going

Was I ever truly happy then?
And what was the general reaction to my addiction?
I no longer know
A dual diagnosis? Self-medication?
MORE liver damage and unwelcome sedation

I needed help and treatment too
My total compliance would be up to you
What prognosis?
Would I need hypnosis?
If I were ever to recover and abstinent stay

From the first day that I learnt about the co-morbidity
I surrendered myself to the medical model's supremacy
In the Max Glatt Unit where for a fortnight I stayed
And learnt of relapse prevention and the Librium regime which I duly obeyed

I slept not too well in those long dark detox nights
Anxiety management had not yet kicked in
The group programmes prevented me from falling from a great height

REFLECTIONS ON LIFE

And day to day I grew in strength and dreamt no longer about London gin

Then came the clinical review and discharge plans
But I was still falling between the great service divide
Alcohol dependence! I even got an ICD code to my name
To make sure that I could never hide the shame
It will never lose its significance

Christopher Ejsmond

Statement

Do you know and feel the dignity of human existence?
What do you see when you wake from your sleep?
How do you declare yourself to the world?
And where do you lay your head when the day is done?

Do you follow the rules of your own making?
What do you feel about those who are faking?
How do you share your dreams with those you love?
And where do you go to nurse the wounds that will not heal?

REFLECTIONS ON LIFE

Stigma

I am not contagious
No need for you to look the other way
Deranged I may be but a friend to you I still remain

Suffer not the ignorance of others' laments and drones
For they forever remain the harbingers of woe
Theirs is the false happiness which locks us others out
And theirs is the misfortune which makes me uneasy in a crowd

Long have I toiled and hidden behind my torments
Suffered too much because of their morbid intents
Why carry on this way, if all else is sound?
Must I forever have my eyes fixed on the ground?

Draw nearer and sit close by me
See how our togetherness can set me free
I have been persecuted far too long and abide in that misery
That stigma brings upon those marginalised from society

All that I ask is for some measure of integration
To bring me back from this unhappy situation
And to cleanse away the stain I do bare
For others in their own way to show that they care

Impose no caveat on how to proceed
Surrender me not to unfriendly company
But stay with me just a little longer

Christopher Ejsmond

While we all learn how to become a little stronger

REFLECTIONS ON LIFE

Surviving

Somehow I managed to survive the worst of it all
Those moments of sadness and emptiness which did call
Upon me in the wilderness years
And nursed me back from this vale of tears

I stood apart from you in those days
Too afraid to ask you to unlodge the darkness of the maze
And yet I went on and followed in tribulation
Alcantara and her dying children

Ask me not for I do not know
How I survived from blow to blow
Surviving is somehow what I am best at
This vessel you see now is stronger than that

Christopher Ejsmond

The Heart

Where there's life there is strife
Where there's life, the surgeons knife
To pierce the wounds of love
And to give way to God above

Where there's blood there is food
A symbiotic thread of gold
The beat of passion in the dark
A promise of tomorrow

To draw us near to the tears of sorrow
To lift us up to the angelic host
Where there's life – make the most
Of every beat, of every beat

REFLECTIONS ON LIFE

The merge

I would like to get to know you better
For you have been like a genie waiting for the day of release
A gift which has lain dormant in the soul for all these years
And now you are back again

I do not know from where you came
But your power I do understand
I recognise you as you recognise me
And your designs to make me a part of you

Forbidden corners which forever remain neglected
And dereliction stands in their way
A building, a room, a bridge
Or any powerful structure such as a water tower or a pylon

These draw me through the energy within
And take hold of me by locking me in
With the electro-magnetic charge of attraction
This is not my world but part of a living death

From here there is no return
And the world of the others who once lived
Is too frightening to let go
And so I communicate with objects from their past

Walking down a deserted street, I am in another era
Not as myself but as another man
And I imagine a world without people

Christopher Ejsmond

A future as real as the past I have known

This power source lasts forever
Merged by that power I live on in an altered state
Though I freeze in motion
And am bereft of any lasting emotion

REFLECTIONS ON LIFE

The other side

In these days that I have wept
God has touched my soul and left
Now I wait for the shackles to fall away
And the shattered splinters to end this day

This pain does not belong to me
Though it's taken everything away
And now I ask the breath of purity
To rescue my soul and restore my sanity

How well I've been caught in the mire
As all around use words which have been used before
A reverse smile transposes itself
So swift to camouflage and redeem its own wealth

I know this is a gift
I've seen it on the other side, as it disappears
Into the ether from which it first endeared
A slave I was right from the start

It grew with me – my closest friend
It set up the rules of this ludicrous game
The winner takes all
And leaves me to nurse the sickness of loss when it ceases to call

The tired shoes are splitting up
And take me to a place to die again
The game is played very carefully
The delicate balance perfects this alliance

Christopher Ejsmond

And YOU, you do what you like
I know you well – you're part of me
Your flowing reality and fluctuations
Describe and encompass me amid strange sensations

You leave me in dereliction
Up and walking but without conviction
You abandon me in this endless roundabout of grief
I lie in your grasp
And does anyone ask me
To get in line that I may wait for your wisdom again to receive

REFLECTIONS ON LIFE

The storm

I stood in the middle of a field
A witness to nature's power
I fell to the ground upon my knees
Full of supernatural breath in that hour

I marvelled upon the spectacle of light
A man reborn in the darkness of night
Rekindled by the majesty and awe
At last I knew what life is for

In a trance I ventured forth
One step at a time – that's all I'm worth
Before Zeus and a host of angels
Safe in their hands as the storm rages

Christopher Ejsmond

The wall

Brick by brick is built the wall
Isolated it stands to menace the fragile mind
To call out and draw me in
To suffocate my identity and my very being

Brick by brick is built the wall
Now alone I stand, part of something greater than myself
Alone and frightened, yet together now WE stand
Still, silent, waiting - like the eye of the storm

Not too long before the winds blow down again
And bring me back to life
Somehow altered, somehow changed
And never to be the way I was before

REFLECTIONS ON LIFE

The Young Ones

The loneliest time of my life was in my teenage years
When the world around me was engulfed in irrational fears
I was ill and needed a true friend
But instead you were all my enemies and me you would not defend
Against the onslaughts of the stronger ones
And of the rebellious and vicious daughters and sons

Instead you pushed me away
Embarrassed by my weakness, you looked to another day
You were never my friends
Your insane laughter meant I could never fully blend
Relief I sought in familial transmission
A Primum Mobile on the road to adulthood's transition

You distanced yourself as the madness took hold of me
A victim of circumstance which I was destined to be
Your empty words rang out like a polluted stream
Of indignant and impatient screams
Mutilated by the silence of others
You wished that I had never been born and that me you could smother

You gave me a bad press at school

Christopher Ejsmond

And you paved the way for me to be everyone's fool
I would still like to know how you got away with it
And rescue the day from your squirming wit
So that I may gracefully go to my death
And savour, on my own terms, one last breath

REFLECTIONS ON LIFE

There are no stars tonight

There are no stars tonight
And no moon to light
The darkness in which we go forth
Weary of battle and the dogs of war

There are no stars tonight
Nothing to bring joy or light
Alone we stand like soldiers on guard
But without an army to command

Christopher Ejsmond

Thursday's Child

Thursday's child has far to go
Speeding through life with nothing to owe
And no-one to see but the face of Jove
Along the well trodden paths of the sacred grove

I was born Thursday's child
Tempestuous, yet meek and mild
A watery grave to call my own
And the sky above which I have known

To distant lands which call my name
I venture forth that I may tame
The celestial parody that is mine to own
And keep by my side where the spirit is sewn

Amid the mottled canopy of the sky above
Where surfaces and boundaries do approve
The silver clouds in their daily dance
And nothing is truly left to chance

When does sadness become depression?
And the bolt out of the blue yields to accession
To agree to the dictate of the day
When yesterday's memories fade away

Now it's autumn and the leaves fall from the trees
Thursday's child has made a plea
To grow wise and in the fullness of time
To look upwards and the golden ladder to climb

REFLECTIONS ON LIFE

Train journey

The sun flickers like a silver mist
Across the carriage that carries me
To the other side of the country
Through rural pastures and foreign cityscapes

To another land
Far beyond the metropolis
Where the sea dwells in perfect harmony
With natural currents and caressing empathy

Bridges swoop and embankments collide
Aboard is the madman who has found a place to hide
Memories begin to fade away
As the dawn brigade lights the way ahead

Confused commuters look on and stare
Not sure what they are seeing or what to say
I am the eternal traveller in their midst
Along life's battered road, I have no cause to protest

My hair is long and my face is drawn
As the wind does blow me from side to side
In this highway to I know not where
And on my return I have no cares

All that I see and hear has a meaning to me
For the stability of otherness has left me
In the speed and rush of the passing train
There is time to dwell on my lasting pain

Christopher Ejsmond

Tribe

The mental health tribe is forged by culture and group identity
We have been assigned a 'sick role' in society
A collective dimension has named us in-valid
As the breakdown of social bonds continues to harm

Social integration has long been the answer
With the tribe comes loss of self and moral guidance
Tribal identity defines and locates us within itself
And places us in the context of the wider world

The fragile social bonds which make us human
Play the social exclusion game and make life feel unreal
Socio-historical and cultural processes at work behind the scenes
Enabled, then disabled by anomie

The distant echo of far way voices and the whispers in the shadows
Move in straight lines along the street
There are deeds to be done and words to be said
And a price to be paid to the past

What chance have you got?
You find out that life's not like that
But the tough times lie ahead
And soon you will drown in your own existence

Life swings around

REFLECTIONS ON LIFE

There's a secret place you must go
To escape from the tribe
That is looking back at you

You cannot resist that which is greater and
stronger
And surely you will wait for the right time
The tribe catches you in its script long before you
are born
It cannot be tamed by wit alone

You got out just in time but you were worse for it
The senses are blunted as you drown in a strange
town
Your new shoes are splitting up
And the sense of guilt is overbearing

Christopher Ejsmond

Unbound

Remove these chains, why don't you?
Please release me and let me go
Think of me in my plight
And surrender me not to eternal night
Illness is not in the mind but in the situation
It confesses all to the prophetic ear
And separates past from present
In a sweep of predictable contingencies
Locked in my world as a child
Playing alone in the garden
Strange sounds all around
And the monotony of life dragging on

Undo the binds that have fallen upon me
And sit by my side as a friend to me
Free me and protect me from adversity
As I look on from the other place
And place my trust in you
To deliver the promise of a life free from doubt
The hum of the motors is persistent
Yet episodic are their invocations
To the other side and the final transmissions
Which harm the sensible souls of this world
And place a burden on their carers
Who one day will restore the world of the bound

REFLECTIONS ON LIFE

Upon Wharncliffe viaduct

I stood one day upon a railway viaduct
In my youth and in the dawn of the second madness
I climbed the forbidden mountainside
And entered a world so tranquil, so beautiful
High above the valley of the Brent
In quest of nature's enigmatic lament

The Egyptian columns my weight did so proudly support
Below, a silver stream and a colony of bats did I see
Their caves were in the hollows
And did they not dwell in the grottoes?
Of this arterial link which had become my refuge
A source of healing and remedy, perhaps

Nature's spectacle danced before me
Symbol and myth entwined for all to see
The unwritten narrative of my life did open
And the source of all wonder and illumination did call
Here I stood, wanderer above the sea of fog
Intuitive protagonist with synthesising primary faculty

In that moment did I realise
That nature's call was a sea of symbolic virtue
A nuance so subtle and fair
On this interior journey to accompany
And recreate a system by which to live
This life and its paradoxical combinations

Christopher Ejsmond

Realms of existence mediate and reconcile
All opposites and duality without
The metaphysical truths of space and time
And the creative powers of the human mind
Unleashed together in my heroic manifesto to the world
Transcending all around in their own spontaneity

The contradiction of man and nature
Of urban and pastoral manifest
And at supernatural behest
I alone was the navigator
And was I not the true creator
Of meaning and the aesthetic imagination?

In trepidation and awe of nature untamed
I strove out to touch the untouchable things
Which had disclosed their existence to me
In ways which taught me to perceive and apprehend again
The subjectivity of all persistence
And to yield once more to remote existence

REFLECTIONS ON LIFE

Watching the trees grow

Sunlight breaks through the leaves
The sky is blue and tender
And an enchanted land beckons
As I watch meaningfully the mystery of creation

A thing of beauty lasts forever
Birds do sing and fly high in the sky
As the clouds drift away
And the rain is frozen and falls no more

The grass on this side is much greener
And rivers do flow faster and cleaner
The texture of the sun on my brow
Takes me to distant lands

I see the golden aura about the shadow of the form
And look both ways, past and future, as the light does dawn
The miracle unfolds and delivers me to the other side
It takes both my hands and leads me on

Time stands still, the moment is now
The labyrinth of the mind spins out of control
And the ephemeral quality of time's passage
Paints a rainbow across the inner sky

The dangers on this road I do know
And there is no safe rite of passage for my return
All is forever moving and changing
In this place where paradise is found

Christopher Ejsmond

I look inward as I look out
And do realise that just as the rose gives honey to the bees
So must I work hard for this state to find again
And take up again the challenge of the few

REFLECTIONS ON LIFE

Weatherman

The weatherman spoke to me the other day on the television screen
How did he know who I was?
And how did he know I was there?
In the relative safety of an armchair

Why did he not utter more?
His words I could not ignore
They were special and meant for me
As he shuffled across the silver screen

The weatherman spoke in riddles and rhyme
Just as I do from time to time
His was a boxed-in world
Mine was one of geometric visions of reality disturbed

What strange stimulus and misinterpretation
Could declare itself to me? Deceitful misinformation
Then, in that moment, I knew that my weary body I sought to dispose
And my suffering mind to repose

Christopher Ejsmond

What vision is left for the man without hope?

What vision is left for the man without hope?
When the sun sets on his sorrows
And he lets pass the promise of all his tomorrows.

What comfort will he find?
In that tortuous bind
To which his soul is confined.

No more is he the master of his own fate
As the demons clamour at the gates of dawn
Must he forever stray blindly among the forlorn?

REFLECTIONS ON LIFE

When the wind blows

When the wind blows
It takes thoughts from inside my head
And delivers them to the passer-by
In the street

When the sun shines
It burns a hole in my head
And blisters my skin
With strange thoughts

When the rain falls
It drowns the sorrows of my heart
And declares freedom
Where there is none

When the sky turns red
It sends a message to my brain
And lingers on in dread
To persecute me with its pain

Christopher Ejsmond

Where I want to be now

Where I want to be
And where I want to go

Is beyond the perimeter
In a forbidden land

Where power and might
Meet heaven and earth
And turn lead into gold
Here is the alchemist at work – behold!

As he spins and turns
Lifeless matter into energy
And dances high above the plateau
Wherein lies the secret afterlife
And brings pleasure to the mind

REFLECTIONS ON LIFE

Whitechapel

On the edge of the city is a place I know
Where in years gone by I used to go
To spend the day in a land which was calling me
And promising to set me free

This is London calling to the far flung suburbs, a city of dreams
On the dusty streets of Petticoat Lane or Stepney Green
Along an artistic route to glorious Whitechapel
I encountered a jolly youth selling his pineapples

In Angel Alley was a Marxist bookstore
Which called me in that I may explore
The secret lives of the East End Jewish radicals
Of their words and deeds to which they were once manacled

How do you measure the immeasurable?
That vast and untold experience so pleasurable?
Of being in another time and place
Where mind and body no longer occupy physical space

The east of the city is the place to be
From this vantage I learnt how to see
With the inner eye of discernment
And the revealed truths of formal judgment

Now that the east has so sweetly spoken
And shown me a world of which nothing is written
I will always carry the truth with me

Christopher Ejsmond

With eyes forever open that I may once again its precious light to see

REFLECTIONS ON LIFE

Who to blame?

I am the answer to the question
That you wish you'd never asked

I'm the lonely soldier
Embattled on the front

Who knows just how much I've suffered
For you in your ignorant bliss?
And who knows what the question was
Which plunged me into eternal abyss?

Christopher Ejsmond

Wild man

I stood that day within a crowd
Entertained and dementedly proud
I entered the soul of them all
And then I began to slip and fall

I fell away, on the other side
No-one around me could abide
I was lost and truly human no more
And those around me marvelled at what they saw

It didn't last long, that frenzied state
Within the space of an afternoon the wildness did abate
But I was left in perpetual daze
And had a found new way to amaze

They tried to help me, to calm me down
But my mind was shattered as I lay still on the ground
To this day I will always remember
That wild man to which I did surrender

REFLECTIONS ON LIFE

You've changed

It used to be so good
But it's different now
Then the other one came
And blew you away
To another day
Where you changed and mutated
Into something new
And something more dangerous than before

At first it was the power of the circle
The great celestial ouroboros devouring my fragile mind
Then came the numbers and letters with which
I strove to put right to the world
Flight was never an option
For the lure of the madness was always great
Odd and even, the number have been
Odd ones giving some relief as the measure of normality

The even ones were never full of delight
For they reduced the dance but negated my very existence
Then came the curse of the electric switch and of things mechanical
Of paths and doorways and the act of reading itself
And looking in a certain way at things
The actors in the absurd play came and went on stage
My mind was like an orchestra without a conductor

Christopher Ejsmond

And all was a massive mental structure which had to be neutralised piece by piece

You have changed over the years but you are still there
I have learnt how to reclaim and retrace some of my own thoughts
From your sickening impositions
And have learnt that no harm comes to those near me
And how to predict the pitfalls
But then the second madness came
And eloped with you while I stood silently by
Drowned in my own sorrows, I learnt how to cry

www.ingramcontent.com/pod-product-compliance
Ingram Content Group UK Ltd.
Pitfield, Milton Keynes, MK11 3LW, UK
UKHW041412180426
11947UKWH00007B/86